Total
Mind-Body-Spirit
Weight Loss

Linda Mackenzie

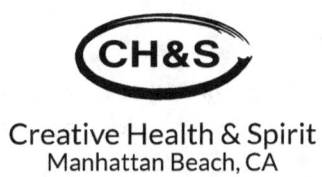

Creative Health & Spirit
Manhattan Beach, CA

Creative Health & Spirit
P.O. Box 385
Manhattan Beach, CA 90267
www.lindamackenzie.net

© **2024 Creative Health & Spirit**

All rights reserved. No part of this book may be reproduced or utilized in any form or by any means, electronic or mechanical, including photocopying, recording or by any information storage and retrieval system, without permission in writing from the publisher.

No part of this publication may be reproduced or transmitted in any form or by any means, electronic or mechanical, including photocopy, recording, or any information storage and retrieval system now known or to be invented, without permission in writing from the publisher, except by a reviewer who wishes to quote brief passages in connection with a review written for inclusion in a magazine, newspaper or broadcast.

Disclaimer: The opinions expressed in this book represent the personal views of the author. The ideas, suggestions and procedures in this book are not intended as a substitute for consulting your health care provider. Individuals with health problems should always see their health care provider before administering any suggestions made in this book. Neither the author nor the publisher is engaged in rendering professional advice and shall not be held liable or responsible for any loss, injury, damage, your specific health or allergy or adverse reactions arising from the information or suggestion in this book. Any application of the materials set forth in the following pages is at the reader's discretion and is his or her sole responsibility.

Library of Congress Control Number: 2023923403

ISBN 979-8-9867179-2-0 (Paperback)
ISBN 979-8-9867179-3-7 (Ebook)
ISBN 979-8-9867179-4-4 (Audiobook)

Printed in the United States

Book design: Clarity Designworks

To send correspondence to the author of this book, mail a first class letter to the author c/o Publisher. Author will be forwarded your letter or contact the author directly at lindamackenzie.com.

As a surgeon helping cancer patients recover from so-called incurable diseases I learned the key to helping people heal are the changes they make in their lifestyles, beliefs and self-esteem. The mind is a powerful tool and when it becomes the positive coach for your body amazing results can occur. Linda and I speak the truth because we care not about the best pill to take but how to live your healthiest and longest life. So get Linda's book and use it as your guide book.

—Bernie Siegel, MD, author of *Love, Medicine & Miracles*

In Linda Mackenzie's new book, *Total Mind-Body-Spirit Weight Loss*, we are given a holistic approach, that not only is effective, but also creative and custom designed for each person. Filled with amazing visualizations, tips, and insights, this book is a MUST READ for anyone who struggles with their weight.

—Sharkie Zartman, author of *Have Fun Getting Fit* and *Shark Sense*

In her book, *Total Mind-Body-Spirit Weight Loss*, Linda has captured the essence of success in dealing with weight management. Her approach harnesses the power of the mind to transcend faulty behaviors through visualization of positive ones, including making the right choices for food intake. This is a must read for anyone ready for a transformative approach in their weight loss journey.

—Dr. Jane Greer, author of *Am I Lying To Myself?*

The Total Mind-Body-Spirit Weight Loss Program beautifully illustrates the power that we each have within us to improve our physical, mental, emotional, and spiritual health. For people who desire to right-size their bodies, this book provides a step-by-step guide to achieving their goal using their ample inner resources.

—Ran D. Anbar, MD, author of *Changing Children's Lives with Hypnosis*

Linda Mackenzie's *Total Mind-Body-Spirit Weight Loss* is a tour-de-force in how to recreate your thoughts, emotions and behavior to control your weight and master your health. She combines mind, body, spirit, nutrition, visualizations and a realm of powerful methods to guide the reader through her program. If you wish to control your weight, or master how your thoughts, feelings and behavior help manifest your life, this book needs to be your handy reference. No home...or kitchen...should be without it.

—Dr. Ron Dalrymple, author of *Mind Games People Play*

*This book is dedicated to my daughter, Lisa,
who is one of the brightest lights in my life.*

....

This program is the culmination of two years of intense research and was originally produced as an AudioVisualization tape series. Most deserving thanks goes to Jill Schettler who said, "Have you ever thought about making your tape series into a book?" It is because of her that this book is in existence. I wish to thank all the authors, writers, doctors, hypnotherapists, naturopaths, fitness trainers and nutrition experts who are too numerous to mention that generously gave me their information and time. My friends and family deserve a big thanks for patiently listening to my ideas. Most of all I want to thank God who always provides my inspiration, boosts my fortitude and consistently cheers me on.

CONTENTS

Preface..ix

Chapter One   Introduction to the Program 1

Chapter Two   Keys to Weight Loss................................. 7

Chapter Three   How and Why Visualization Works.................. 13

Chapter Four   Commitment to Weight Loss 19
                      Mind-Body-Spirit Integration Visualization 22

Chapter Five   Mind Transformation 29
                      Altering Emotional Ties to Eating Visualization 31

Chapter Six   Body Transformation............................. 39
                      Changing Eating Habits Visualization 41

Chapter Seven   Exercise Motivation 49
                      Exercise Visualization............................... 52

Chapter Eight   Stress Relieving Meditations 59
                      Stress Visualizations:
                      "The Waterfall" 62
                      "The Ocean" 65
                      "The Healing Pool" 67

Chapter Nine   Thin Meditations................................ 69
                      Thin Visualizations:
                      "The Downward Staircase" 71
                      "The Weight Loss Sauna"........................... 75
                      "The Perfect Body"................................. 78

Epilogue 81

Bonus Section   'LindaMac' Diet................................. 83

PREFACE

Weight Loss is a big issue. Almost everyone at some time in their lives has wanted to lose weight. Yet most of the programs out there work only on the body and ignore the mind and spirit. As a Doctoral Clinical Hypnotherapist Candidate and Psychic, I help people reach their physical, emotional and spiritual goals. After helping thousands of people through my private and group hypnotherapy sessions, lectures and my radio show I believe that manifestation of any goal must combine the mind, body and spirit together to effect a lasting change.

For many years people have been asking me to come up with a weight loss program. Weight Loss is not an easy issue since everyone is an individual and the way they gain and lose weight are as individualized as they are. So this project became a very serious task for me. First, because when I develop a self-empowerment tool it must be simple and be able to work for a majority of people. Second, I was an engineer for 18 years and my left brain will not allow me to overlook detail. I talked to many experts and people nationwide. People who were successful with weight loss and those who were not. For two years I researched. I was looking for the common threads. What was it that was similar in every case? Why did 97 out of 100 people who diet regain the weight back in less than a year? What ties these threads together?

My left brain cataloged the details and my right brain finally found the answer (with a little Divine Guidance for I'm sure that God looked down one day and thought, "She's still working on that? Let me send her a little help!"). STRESS is the common thread. I found that there are four types of stress that cause or contribute to weight gain: Emotional. Physical. Environmental. Nutritional. Everything that affects weight gain falls under one of these categories. Chapter One of this book defines this in more detail.

By eliminating or minimizing stress on these four levels people can lose weight and keep it off for life. Commitment also plays a key role. If a person is not committed they will not be motivated. No motivation—No weight loss. I had found the threads. Now how do I tie them together to self-empower people to lose weight?

Back to the left brain. Back to the "I knows." I know that visualization works because I cured myself of a severe chronic illness using visualization and diet. I know there are several hypnosis methods used to effect weight loss—but not every method works for everyone. I know people assimilate information through one or more of these methods visual, audio and tactile or touch. I know that the types and amounts of stress differs daily for each person. There were hundreds of these I knows and lots of research hours put in to get the "I knows." My left brain sorted through the information, my right brain balanced the pros and cons and Divine Intervention guided the whole process.

Finally the Program was complete. It works. Just being immersed in the process of creating this program was effective in weight loss. I lost 8 lbs. which was not my intention. This in itself is amazing because intention is one of the most important parts of visualization. Yet the program worked. It's funny how God always helps me walk my talk.

My field tests have realized fantastic results. The patients were between 20-150 lbs. overweight. I told them not to exercise and not to change their eating habits. Ha! Because of the Visualizations they all did some form of exercise—they couldn't help themselves. They all leaned towards eating healthy food. In less than 2 months one girl had dropped 2 dress sizes; in 6 weeks another had dropped 22 lbs., another 5 lbs. and the results went on and on.

The visualizations are powerful. They are designed to use what you need, when you need them. Visualization usually takes six weeks to work and should be done in the morning and at night. You may see results before six weeks, but if you don't keep at it. It will work.

The funny thing that I didn't expect to happen was that everyone said they were not only losing weight but they were happier. The stress in their lives was being reduced and they felt so relaxed they were enjoying life. They reported feeling centered and whole in body, mind and spirit. One man, who didn't need to lose weight, plays the tapes for stress reduction.

What a joy to know I have created a tool for someone to help themselves. For only with self-empowerment can people positively change themselves and make their way to their next step on their special path in life. My mission in life is to "Light the Way with Energy, God and Love" and to help at least one person a day. I am so glad that with this publication that I can reach many people who will be helped on many levels.

So after a long, hard road filled with determination and persistence the Program is ready. I believe that you are ready too! Good luck to you. I know you will lose the weight you need.

—Linda Mackenzie

CHAPTER ONE

INTRODUCTION TO THE PROGRAM

- ∞ How To Use This Program
- ∞ Why Stress Causes Weight Gain
- ∞ The Six Tips To Success

Welcome to The Total Mind-Body-Spirit Weight Loss Program. This Program is designed to give you mind control for weight control. Using the visualization methods in this book you will be given the tools to be able to lose the weight you want and keep it off for life. The visualizations are designed so that you can use each one over and over as you need them. You are unique and after reading the book once you will know how often and which visualizations to use to reach your goal. Don't worry you'll know! Visualization is a powerful tool to help you access your mind-body connection. Visualization DOES Work! Have no doubt about that. The Olympic Teams and many professional athletes use visualization successfully to improve their performance as you will now do to improve your health and appearance. Be assured that this Program has everything you need for successful weight loss and that you will lose weight.

In this chapter you will discover why stress is the major culprit to weight gain and what you can do about this. In Chapter 2 you will be given the Nutritional keys to maximize and customize a weight loss program that's right for your body. For faster weight loss a discussion about dietary supplements and herbs is provided. Since visualization is the primary method used in this book, Chapter 3 will explain how and why visualization works and how to access your mind-body connection to lose the weight you want without effort. You will even learn how to prepare for a visualization. So sit back, relax and let's start losing weight!

Did you know that of people who diet 97 out of 100 will regain the weight within the 1st year and that the majority of people who diet will regain fat faster than before they started dieting? These are staggering facts that you may already know. However most people don't know that stress is the major culprit to weight gain.

Let me explain. There are four types of stress that affect how we look, think and feel. There is Nutritional Stress when the body isn't getting the right foods, supplements and nutrients. Emotional Stress that creates emotional ties to eating. Physical Stress where your body is not getting enough exercise or when your body's systems are out of balance. Last there is Environmental Stress or inside and outside factors that can contribute to your body's weight gain.

Type of Stress	Why	How it Affects Weight Gain
Nutritional	Not Enough Right Nutrient	Body Does Not Process Food Correctly
Emotional	Eating for the "Wrong Reasons"; "Holding On" to Weight	Body/Mind Help Develop Cravings; Food Dependency, Overeating
Physical	Not Enough Exercise	Slows Body Metabolism; Increases Fat Storage
Environmental	Outside Pollutants; Food Pollutants	Slows Down Food and Other Body Processes

To effectively lose weight we need to attack all levels of stress and learn to minimize this stress every day in our lives. Now how do we really lose weight?

Here are Six Essential Tips that are needed for successful weight loss

First, you need to make a commitment to lose weight. Not with just your mind, but with your body and spirit as well. A Total Commitment On All Levels! In Chapter Four, *Commitment to Weight Loss and the Mind-Body-Spirit Integration Visualization,* we address this issue. In the visualization you will learn the reasons why you gain weight on a mind and body level and integrate that with your spirit or desire level. You will gain self-acceptance on who you are meant to be and acquire the motivation to lose the weight you need and want.

But most important you will gain a REAL COMMITMENT TO WEIGHT LOSS ON A MIND-BODY- SPIRIT LEVEL that will make you FEEL, KNOW and TRUST that the weight you want to lose will be gone and you will be able to keep it off for Life!

Second you need to transform your mind to decrease Emotional Stress. With Chapter 5, *Mind Transformation and the Altering Emotional Ties to Eating Visualization,* you will learn to harness the power of thinking thin.You will also be able to release negative behavior patterns that have inhibited you from losing weight and eliminate negative thinking. Finally you will *naturally* reduce your food intake *without effort.*

Third, you need to change your eating habits. In Chapter Six, *Body Transformation and Changing Your Eating Habits Visualization,* will increase your nutritional awareness and change your eating habits to ones that are healthy for you. You'll automatically select the foods that are right for you, control bad eating habits and overeating without cravings or hunger. You'll envision who you are at your ideal weight and begin to make that image a reality.

Fourth, you need to get exercise. Chapter Seven, *Exercise Motivation and Exercise Visualization,* helps you find the right exercise for your body and motivates you to exercise regularly. You'll experience joy every time you exercise so that you make your body feel as good as it looks.

Fifth, you need to release the stress in your life. With Chapter Eight, *Stress Relieving Visualizations,* you will be able to cope with and release all levels of stress to keep your commitment to lose weight and be able to maintain a positive attitude.

Sixth, which is most important, you need to Think Thin to Be Thin. Using Chapter 9, *Thin Visualizations,* you will be able to maintain and keep your weight off. You can even use them daily to boost your body to lose weight faster.

So to put it simply—To get the body you want—you need a strong commitment, the right attitude, the right foods, the right exercise and you need to reduce stress. Don't worry. This book will help you with all this.

HOW TO USE THIS PROGRAM

The visualizations in this book will access your mind-body connection to reduce nutritional, physical, emotional and environmental stress. You are unique so what you need to do to lose weight is unique. The visualizations are designed so that you can use what you need when you need them. Read the book through once and do the visualizations in order. Then decide which visualizations you need for each day. Do one or all depending on whatever you need. I suggest you do at least one of the following: Mind-Body-Spirit Integration, Altering Emotional Ties to Eating or Changing Eating Habits **AND** at least one Stress and one Thin visualization a day. Use them as often as you need to keep committed, motivated and losing weight.

Visualization should be done in the morning and before bedtime for at least six weeks. You should see and feel results before the six weeks. In fact some people have reported weight loss the very next day. If this happens—Great! If it doesn't be patient. IT WILL WORK!

CHAPTER TWO

KEYS TO WEIGHT LOSS

- ∞ 8 Nutritional Keys
- ∞ Nutritional Vitamins and Supplements
- ∞ Nutritional Herbs

These nutritional keys will open the door to your weight loss. These keys can maximize your success. By using them in conjunction with the visualizations, you will have permanent weight loss, feel full of energy and attain your ideal weight faster without strict diets, terrible struggles or tremendous effort.

Key 1 — Don't Skip Meals, Eat Smaller Meals

If you eat smaller meals every 2-3 hours it will decrease the cortisone, cholesterol and insulin levels in your body. Why is this important? Because it will decrease fat storage in your body. When you skip a meal cortisone levels rise and burn muscle tissue and not the fat that you need to lose *and* the pancreas secretes more insulin which actually increases body fat. Remember if you starve your body and then eat large meals the extra food is stored as fat in your body.

> *So Remember Key 1:*
> *Don't Skip Meals, Eat Smaller Meals Every 2-3 Hours*

Key 2 — Choose the Right Foods

A low fat, high fiber diet comprised of mostly vegetables, whole grains, legumes and fruits will slow down your digestion, absorb food better and steady blood sugar levels in your body. This makes the body work more efficiently and helps reduce or eliminate cravings. Eating mostly raw foods is also good for your body. Some foods can even slow down your body's metabolism such as sugars and fats.

Limit dairy products which are high in animal fats. Avoid sugar, salt, white flour, white rice, coffee, soda, alcohol, artificial flavorings and coloring, and food preservatives. Kelp can help normalize thyroid metabolism.

Avoid partially hydrogenated oils (e.g. margarine, vegetable shortening and salad oils). These oils have a negative effect on our body's cardiovascular, reproductive and hormonal systems. They effect our metabolism and liver functions. But most important these partially hydrogenated oils actually change the size, number and composition of our fat cells. Replace these hydrogenated oils with Omega 3 and GLA Fatty Acids such as Flaxseed Oil, Olive Oil, Borage Oil, Wheat Germ Oil or Evening Primrose Oil. These oils have body rejuvenating qualities and *increase* your metabolism and *decrease* fluid retention. Remember the body needs some fat to enable our immune system to fight disease—so a low fat diet is better for you than a no-fat diet.

So Remember Key 2: Eat the Right Foods

Key 3 — Build Lean Muscle Tissue

Lean muscle tissue burns 5X as many calories as other body tissue. If you start a resistance training exercise program, such as weight lifting, for 3 times a week, 30 minutes a day you will lose weight and not have to reduce your calorie intake. Any exercise is important, so find one you like and do it regularly. Not only does exercise help you lose weight but it helps premature aging and helps fight disease. It helps to prevent osteoporosis, heart disease and stroke, just to name a few.

So Remember Key 3: Build Lean Muscle Tissue

Key 4 — Drink Water

Drinking 3 quarts of water a day suppresses your appetite. It helps get rid of body toxins and allows the liver to process more fat. Drinking 1 gallon of water a day burns 300 calories which is equivalent to running 3 miles.

So Remember Key 4- Drink Water

Key 5 — Fat Burning Vitamins, Minerals, Supplements and Herbs

There are many vitamins, minerals, supplements and herbs that help you lose weight. Remember to check with your doctor, nutritionist or alternative medicine practitioner to find the right ones for you. Here are a some to check out:

Start with the right vitamins, preferably from a health food store so that they can be digested and absorbed. Some of the over the counter vitamins do not get past the liver into your system and are even found only partially digested in your intestines. There are also differences in vitamins. There are natural vitamins and synthetic vitamins. Natural vitamins are derived from plants and animals and their basic natural structure is maintained. Synthetic vitamins are laboratory manufactured. Some synthetic vitamins can be identical in molecular structure and activity as the natural vitamins, such as Vitamin C and Vitamin B. However, some vitamins cannot be identically duplicated (e.g. Vitamin E) so natural vitamins should be preferred because they absorb into the body better.

All minerals are natural. There are Chelated Minerals that are attached to protein molecules to increase the absorption rate in the body. These usually have a two part name ending in -ate (like Chromium Picolinate). Collodial Minerals are suspended in liquid, usually water, and may be even better absorbed by the body than chelated minerals. To select the right vitamins and minerals for you, ask your health food store, Nutritionist or Doctor to help you.

Super Foods like blue-green algae, wheat grass and barley grass can increase your metabolism and raise the energy levels in the body. These SuperFoods are full of vitamins, minerals, enzymes and protein. They contain chlorophyll which is an important, powerful nutrient. Super Foods are also one of the best body detoxifiers. It helps flush the liver and purify the blood.

Supplements and Enzymes can help you to lose weight. L-Carnitine is a fat burner. L-Glutamine helps to reduce cravings and builds muscle tissue. L-Argnine is also a muscle builder. Chitosan is a fat absorber. Lecithin helps water retention. Chromium Picolinate helps to burn fat and balance blood sugar levels in the body. Betaine Hydrochloride or Papaya Enzymes help digest protein, such as meat, out of the body faster. There are so many and these are just a few. Check with your health food store or nutritionist for the ones that are right for you.

Detoxification and elimination of foods from the body is very important to weight loss. Acidolphilus and Colon Cleansers help the body's elimination and detoxification and gets the body to run more efficiently.

Many herbs such as kola nut, ginseng, astralgulus and licorice root can help you lose weight. Peppermint, fennel, basil, bay leaves, caraway and clove aid digestion and green tea is excellent for rejuvenation. Some fluid retention herbs are: buchu, coriander, uva ursi, juniper and cornsilk. There are so many herbs that can help with weight loss that a book probably could be written about this subject. Even certain spices can help increase metabolism and weight loss. Here are some:

Ginger, cayenne pepper and mustard increases metabolism; cinnamon, bay leaf and clove control blood sugar levels and help to diminish cravings.

So Remember Key 5:
Fat Burning Vitamins, Minerals, Supplements and Herbs

Key 6 — Avoid Toxins

To get your body to run more efficiently, cut out caffeine and alcohol. Please note that tea has more caffeine than coffee. Watch your drugs, some "street drugs", over the counter and prescription drugs can cause side effects of weight gain.

So Remember Key 6: Avoid Toxins

Key 7 — Get Adequate Sleep and Treat Yourself

Adequate sleep reduces stress and allows your body to store more energy for the next day. Remember to be nice to yourself. You deserve it. Why not get a massage. Not only does it relieve stress but massage also helps circulation, gets rid of body toxins and aids many systems in the body.

Remember Key 7: Get Adequate Sleep and Treat Yourself

Key 8 — Use Visualization

This will keep you on track and is a real major key to weight loss. Visualization uses positive images to stimulate emotions that cause physical reactions in the body. It helps to access your mind-body connection to help you manifest whatever you want—including weight loss.

So Remember Key 8: Use Visualization

CHAPTER THREE

HOW AND WHY VISUALIZATION WORKS

- ∞ How to Access the Mind-Body Connection
- ∞ Why Keeping Positive Works
- ∞ What and Why Is Intention Important
- ∞ How to Prepare for a Visualization

Visualization is one of the most important parts of this book. It's how you reach your spirit or desire. You'll lose the weight you want if you are dedicated and use the hints and visualizations in this book. In this chapter you will learn how to access the mind-body connection and discover why keeping positive is very effective to weight loss. You'll even find out how important intention is and how intention relates to you for losing your weight. At the end of this chapter you will find out how to prepare for a visualization and this method is used with all the visualizations in this book.

You *can* manifest anything you want in life with Visualization, including weight loss. Visualization works and here's why. It has been proven that there is a mind-body connection. Visualization accesses this connection and allows you to discover your own resources to help you lose weight.

What is Visualization?
Visualization uses positive images to help you accomplish your weight loss.

How do you Access the Mind-Body Connection?
The mind is this—The mental form of the mind is emotion and emotion produces a feeling. The body's physical form is sensation. When we get an emotion it produces a feeling that turns into a physical sensation. Here's an example: You're watching a scary movie, you get frightened and then you get goose bumps on your body.

Visualization uses positive images that produce feelings (e.g. you are committed to weight loss) and this turns into physical sensations in your body that manifests the weight loss.

How does Visualization work?
Let's take a look at the brain. It is divided into 2 sides: The Left, Logical side where our logic, words and rational thought comes from and the

Right, Creative side which is where our intuition and our imagination is. Normally we are in a left, logical brain mode but when we yield to our right brain or creative side we actually balance the brain and access the mind-body connection which allows us to make the changes we need to achieve our goal.

We are what we Think! So Think Positive. It is interesting to note that negative emotions lower our immune system, keeps us bogged down mentally and makes it harder to change. Having negative emotions delays us from reaching our goals and actually stops us from getting what we want. Many recent studies show that Positive emotions boost our immune system and makes the brain work in a balanced mode. This balanced mode is better for accepting and making changes. It actually helps us attain our weight loss goal.

Let's take a moment to clarify how thinking positive actually affects success. Over a period of time by replacing negative thoughts with positive ones you can change your belief system. Changing your belief systems helps to propel you to success. You must BELIEVE you will lose the weight. To help you believe and manifest positive thought you need to incorporate it in your life. Try focusing on the positive things in your life whenever you get a negative thought. Try reading inspirational books or associate with positive people and inspirational groups. Positive thinking brings endless possibilities. Negative thinking eliminates possibilities. Shifting to positive thought whenever negative ones appear will help you change the way you process your thoughts and ultimately positive thinking will become a normal response in your life.

You will ultimately become more joyful and reach any goal easier. It really is your responsibility to succeed because if you are successful it helps to motivate other people. If other people are motivated the world becomes a positive, happier place. You can succeed with positive thought.

How do we Keep Positive and Balance the Brain?

We can't keep positive if we live in the past or the future. This keeps our minds fragmented and out of focus with what we want to accomplish. You can't do anything about the past—it's over. You can't do anything about the future because there are too many variables. We need to forget the past and the future and learn to deal with Now—This Moment. When we learn to live in the moment in a Go with the Flow Mode it allows us to be more receptive and accept change. When we accept change, changes happen easier. We *do* set up loose goals and then put the INTENTION of what we want to accomplish to work. We also cannot try to set rigid goals, try to control situations or outcomes, set expectations, be negative in our thinking or be egotistical with our intention because this creates a Paradox or contradiction in the brain. Let me try to explain this. Have you ever wanted something so much and it doesn't happen and then when you don't want it—it happens? Well that's the Paradox. The more you desire the results the more the results won't happen. It's doesn't seem fair but this is a reality on how the brain works. So we can't focus on the results—we need to focus on the Intention.

How do we put the Intention of Losing Weight to Work?

First what is Intention?

    Intention is not trying to control the outcome—" I will lose weight!"

    Intention is not negative thinking—"I'll never lose weight!"

    Intention is not the ego—" I can make myself lose weight!"

    Intention is not setting up expectations or goals—"Tomorrow I will lose the weight."

**INTENTION OF LOSING WEIGHT IS
TO FEEL, KNOW AND TRUST
THAT YOUR WEIGHT LOSS IS BEING ACCOMPLISHED!**

Remember our body, mind and spirit are working 24 hours a day, 365 days a year to manifest what we want. That's it's job. So feel, trust and know this.

Visualization is a great method that puts our Intention to work and this method works for anything, not just weight loss!

How do we Prepare for a Visualization?

1. Define your intention—Be specific

2. Find a quiet place where you won't be disturbed.

3. Get calm and focused.

4. Keep your eyes open or closed, whatever you prefer.

5. Concentrate on the breath and breathing deeply. This activates the Vagus nerve which runs from the medulla in the brain and down to the base of the spine. It then branches out to the lungs, heart and intestinal tract. The Vagus Nerve is the major quieting nerve in the body. When we focus on the breath and breathe deeply it always lowers blood pressure and the heart, respiratory and pulse rate.

6. Relax, continue breathing and do the specific visualization.

The first time you start the visualizations in this book, please do them in chapter order. Then decide which visualization you need to do daily. Do one visualization from a chapter or all of them. Whatever you feel you need. I suggest you do at least 1 stress meditation and at least one thin meditation a day along with any visualization that you feel is necessary to keep you committed, motivated and losing weight.

Visualization should be done in the morning and at bedtime. It takes about six weeks to get the full effect but you should see and feel results before that. Some people feel results the very first time, some people experience weight loss after the very first day. If you don't, be patient. It will work.

Remember to Live in the Now, Keep Positive and FEEL, KNOW and TRUST that you are losing the weight and you will! You're on your Road to Weight Loss!

I know you will lose weight. I hope you enjoy the tapes and I wish you Purpose, Patience and Peace.

CHAPTER FOUR

COMMITMENT TO WEIGHT LOSS

- ∞ Reach a Real Commitment on All Levels

- ∞ Learn Why You "Hold On" to Weight

- ∞ Gain Motivation and Self-Acceptance

You might ask why your mind-body and spirit need to be integrated to lose weight. Well losing weight is not a spectator sport. It requires a commitment on all levels. Our physical bodies need the right foods, supplements and exercise. On a mental level we need to release negative emotional problems and mental processes that keep our weight on. Our spirit or desire to lose weight is very important. With the various stresses that come into our lives every day we need to keep our body, mind and spirit constantly motivated. Without a solid commitment you can't stay motivated. Most times the reasons why a commitment is ineffective is that we make a commitment on just one level. For example, you think that diet alone will be enough to manifest the change or you make a mental commitment and don't follow through by adjusting your body to healthy eating habits. By integrating the commitment on the mind-body-spirit levels you gain cooperation with all parts of you. Your whole self participates on all levels. There isn't any part of you that is left out of the process, so it has to work.

We may not even know why we gain weight on a conscious level or in fact which level or combination of levels are responsible for "Holding On" to the weight. Let me give you some examples. Some Psychics and Healers are overweight because in their work they expend more energy on a physical and spiritual level than the normal person. They compensate by ingesting food or sugar to restore their energy. They may not even be aware they are doing this. Sometimes a physical experience of past child abuse will shift the mind to eating to make the victim unattractive as a protection mechanism. There are unique reasons for each person. Some are conscious, some are sub-conscious but they are there. These reasons no matter what they are make it hard to maintain a commitment and motivation to lose weight and contributes to keeping the weight on.

By determining the reasons, then acknowledging that they are there helps the acceptance process and opens the door to success. All you have to do then is step through that door. Don't worry about releasing the reasons. Right now we want to establish a REAL commitment on a mind-body-spirit level. The subsequent chapters in this book will deal with releasing the reasons on each level.

In the following visualization you will learn the hidden reasons why you retain weight, gain self-acceptance, acquire motivation to lose the weight you want and most important

> REACH A REAL COMMITMENT TO WEIGHT LOSS
> ON A MIND-BODY-SPIRIT LEVEL.

So sit back, relax and get ready to start to lose your weight!

MIND-BODY-SPIRIT INTEGRATION VISUALIZATION

Intention: To Make a Total Commitment to Weight Loss

Find a comfortable place where you won't be disturbed and sit in a comfortable chair. Now sit back and relax with both feet on the floor and place your hands on the arm rests of the chair or in your lap—whichever is comfortable for you. Start to breathe very deeply and concentrate on the breath and breathing. Concentrate as you breathe deeply letting the air come into your nose and out your mouth. Concentrate and breathe IN with the nose and OUT with the mouth. IN with the nose and OUT with the mouth. IN with the nose and OUT with the mouth. Now let's concentrate on breathing OUT with the mouth and IN with the nose. And OUT with the mouth and IN with the nose. And OUT with the mouth and IN with the nose...

Imagine you are in a large open field. The sky is the most beautiful blue you have ever seen. There are a few soft, puffy clouds floating by and the sun is shining. The temperature is exactly right for you. You are feeling so relaxed. Look at the green grass. Smell the flowers that dot the field. Hear the birds singing around you. Feel a gentle breeze caress your body as you start to feel more relaxed than you have ever known yourself to be. Look up at the sun and feel it's warmth. Raise your hands up to the sun and feel it's warmth surround you. Now watch as the rays of sunlight come out of the sun and into your fingertips. Feel the warmth as the rays enter into your fingertips and go inside your body. Watch and feel the rays of the sun as they travel through your body. Gently, softly entering your body. Feel the rays of the sun go to your neck. Your shoulders. Your back. We seem to hold so much tension here. Now watch as the rays grow brighter and brighter. Feel the warmth as the rays gently melt and absorb all the stress in your neck. Your shoulders. Your back. Leaving you feeling so relaxed. So peaceful and so very, very relaxed. Now watch as the rays go to every stress spot in your body- relieving the tension, melting the tension, absorbing the tension. making you feel so very relaxed. So very peaceful. Eliminating all pain. Making you feel deeper and deeper relaxed. More relaxed than you've ever known yourself to be. The rays absorbing emotional stress, physical stress. Just melting it away. Feel the tension just melt away from every organ, every fiber, every tissue and every bone in your body. Just melting away. Now feeling more relaxed than you've ever known yourself to be—watch and feel as the rays come out of your body the same way they went in, taking all the stress, all the tension, all the pain out of the body leaving you stress free and so very, very relaxed.

To your right you see a path. Turn and walk down this path. As you walk down the path, to your left you see some trees. These trees are beautiful. They have silver trunks and many tiny golden metal leaves. See how the golden leaves glint in the sun. Hear how the leaves softly tinkle in the soft gentle breeze. You are so peaceful here.

So relaxed. As you walk through the trees you see a beautiful grassy area. Sunlight is peeking through the trees and as you sit down in this grassy area you see a pond with a waterfall. It is so peaceful here.

You are so relaxed. Hear the birds singing and the leaves of the trees tinkling in the breeze. Hear the gentle flowing of the waterfall. What a peaceful spot. You are very relaxed and comfortable here. This is a safe place. Your private place.

There is no judgment, no goals, no expectations. Just Being here in this moment. You are a watcher, an observer. No negative feelings can touch you here. No pain. You are merely Observing. Watching. Look to your left and watch as the part of you that is your physical body comes towards you. There is no judgment. You are just watching, listening, observing. Watch as your physical body sits down next to you. Listen as it tells you the reasons that are stopping it from losing weight. You may not be able to hear all the words but know that you are absorbing this information. There is no judgment. You are safe. Listen and observe. Listen as your physical body tells you what it needs to lose weight. about the foods it needs, the exercise. Everything that it needs to lose the weight. Listen.

(Close your eyes for a moment and Listen. Listen.)

When your physical body is done thank your physical body for giving you the information on what it needs. You understand and know that everything you need to do to help your physical body accomplish it's goal to lose weight will automatically be done. Without effort. Tell your physical body that you understand and accept what it needs to be whole and healthy. Smile at your physical body and watch as it smiles back. You feel the trust blossoming between you. Knowing you share the same goal to be the best that you can be. To be whole and healthy in body. Feel the acceptance, the cooperation, the love between you and your physical body. You feel, know and trust that you are manifesting your ideal body right now, in this time, in this place. As you and your physical body sit in the sun feeling so very, very relaxed on the soft green grass.

Now watch as your mental body comes slowly walking towards you and your physical body. There is no judgment, no goals, no expectations. You are merely watching. Observing. Listening. Watch as your mental body sits down next to you. Listen as your mental body tells you what is stopping it from losing weight.

You may not be able to hear all the words but know that you are absorbing all the information. There is no judgment. You are safe. Listen and observe. Listen as your mental body tells you what it needs to lose weight. About the Emotional Issues, the Mental Processes. Everything that it needs to lose the weight. Listen.

(Close your eyes for a moment and Listen. Listen.)

As you and your physical body listen to your mental body you both understand and know that everything you need to do to help your mental body accomplish it's goal to lose weight will automatically be done. Without effort. When your mental body is done, tell your mental body that you understand and accept what it needs to be whole and healthy. Smile at your mental body and watch as it smiles back. Watch as your physical body tells your mental body that it understands and accepts what it needs. You feel the trust, the knowing that you all share the same goal to be the best that you can be. To be whole and healthy in body, mind and spirit.

Now watch as you all stand up and smile at each other and take each others hands. Feel the acceptance, the cooperation, the love between all of you. You feel, know and trust that your commitment to manifest your ideal body is being done right now, in this time, in this place. As you and your physical body and your mental body smile at each other and stand in the sun feeling so very, very happy and relaxed. Feel the commitment to take care of each other. To know and do what's right for each other without effort. You are happy and at peace knowing your goal of being totally committed to losing weight is being accomplished.

Now watch as your physical body comes over to you and holds you. Feel the love. The sameness of purpose as you feel your physical body melt into you. Feel yourself getting stronger, being committed. Feel the love permeate your being. Watch as your mental body comes over to you and holds you. Feel the sameness of purpose, the commitment as your mental body melts into you. Feeling stronger. Feeling balanced. Feeling centered. Feeling Wholeness.

Feel the trust and love permeating your being. Resonating within you. You feel whole and at peace In This Time, In This Place, Right Now.

Listen as the golden leaves in the trees tinkle in the breeze. See the sun reflecting in off the golden leaves and watch as a golden light surrounds your body. Sealing you. Making you one in body, mind and spirit. Protecting this feeling of being centered and whole and fully committed to your goal. Feel the commitment within you. Feel the knowing that you will lose the weight and manifest the person you are meant to be. Let's walk back through the trees and back to the field. Look up at the sun and raise your hands. Give thanks for the healing that has taken place today. Smile knowing you are one with yourself and that you will truly accomplish your goal. Feel the Trust. The Joy. The Happiness. Feel the Total Commitment. This Feeling will stay with you.

Take a few moments and continue breathing in and out slowly and when you're ready, go to the next chapter.

CHAPTER FIVE

MIND TRANSFORMATION

- ∞ Release Negative Behavior Patterns
- ∞ Reduce Food Intake Naturally
- ∞ Alter Emotional Ties to Eating

Everyone is unique and people overeat and gain weight for different reasons. No one is the same. However you are personally responsible for putting the weight on and you are personally responsible for taking it off. As you control yourself, your weight will also be controlled. Usually there are emotional reasons why you "hold on" to the weight. It may be because of negative things that have happened in the past, low self-esteem, fear of intimacy with others or even as a control over others. There are so many different emotional reasons that cause emotional stress and this emotional stress can trigger negative eating patterns. By releasing negative emotional ties to eating you will lose weight. In this visualization you will learn the power of thinking thin and release negative behavior patterns that are stopping you from losing weight. You will learn to stop negative thinking and naturally reduce your food intake without effort. But most important you will feel self-confident, alter your emotional ties to eating and start losing the weight you want. So Sit back, Relax and Get Ready to Lose Weight!

ALTERING EMOTIONAL TIES TO EATING VISUALIZATION

Intention: To Alter Emotional Ties To Eating

Find a comfortable place where you won't be disturbed and sit in a comfortable chair. Now sit back and relax with both feet on the floor and place your hands on the arm rests of the chair or in your lap—whichever is comfortable for you. Start to breathe very slowly, very deeply and concentrate on the breath and breathing. Concentrate as you breathe deeply letting the air come into your nose and out your mouth. Concentrate and breathe IN with the nose an OUT with the mouth. IN with the nose and OUT with the mouth. And IN with the nose and OUT with the mouth. Now let's concentrate on breathing slowly OUT with the mouth and IN with the nose. And OUT with the mouth and IN with the nose. And OUT with the mouth and IN with the nose........

Imagine you are sitting in a room. The walls are painted in your favorite color. The chair is so very, very comfortable for you. You are feeling relaxed and so very peaceful. In front of you is a fireplace. The fire is burning brightly and you are warm and cozy. You feel calm and relaxed. As you look into the fire you see so many pretty colors and hear the crackling of the wood. You can smell the wood burning and it is so aromatic and sweet and pungent at the same time. So peaceful. So relaxed.

Feeling the warmth of the fire. Calmly sitting and thinking no thoughts at all. You are just peaceful and serene and so very, very relaxed. Now imagine as your sitting by the fire that the warmth of the fire reaches your toes. It feels so soothing as it enters each and every one of your toes and gradually spreads into your feet. This warm and pleasant sensation. Feel this sensation spread up the ankles and into the legs releasing any tension, any pain just making you very, very relaxed as the warmth spreads throughout your legs and into your pelvic area and up into your abdominal and into your chest muscles. So warm. So soothing.

So peaceful, this warm sensation releasing tension and pain as it continues into your shoulders and down your arms until it reaches your hands. Take a moment and feel this warm sensation reach into every fingertip and now traveling back up the arm and into your shoulders and neck area. We hold so much tension in our neck and shoulders and you feel it just release as this warm soothing sensation releases this tension. Tension just oozing away making you feel so relaxed. So very, very relaxed. Now feel the warmth go up through the neck and into your face and your head and down your spinal column branching out to the back and into all your organs. And now all parts of your body are warm and relaxed by this warm soothing sensation. Every organ, every fiber, every tissue, every bone in your body is so very, very relaxed.

Now get up out of the chair keeping this relaxed feeling with you and turn to your right. At the end of the hall is an open door. Go through the door and walk through and you see a staircase going down to another level. The staircase is covered in your favorite colored carpet.

Let's walk down these stairs slowly and as we walk down each of the ten steps you will feel more relaxed than you have ever known yourself to be. Let's go down now.

Step 10 – Feeling relaxed.

Step 9 – Deeper relaxed.

Step 8 – Feeling safe.

Step 7 – Even deeper.

Step 6 – Doing so very, very well.

Step 5 – Deeper and deeper.

Step 4 – Deeper, Deeper and Deeper.

Step 3 – So Very, Very Relaxed.

Step 2 – Deeper, Deeper and Even Deeper.

At the next step you will be more relaxed than you have ever known yourself to be .... Step 1.

At the bottom of the stair there is a door to your left. Open the door and walk into the room. It is a comfortable room and on one side there is a chair with a bookcase in front of it. These are magic books which will be able to tell you all the reasons that you are emotionally tied to eating. Select a book and sit down in the chair.

The book you have selected is exactly right for you. Open the book and start reading. You may not be able to see the words but know that the information that you need is being absorbed. Just relax and read the book. It tells you why you no longer have to overeat. You have no desire to overeat. As you read, all your emotional ties to eating are just going away. Releasing as the words are being absorbed. All the emotional blocks just seem to melt away. They just disappear. Each and every one.

(Close your eyes for a moment and feel the information being absorbed.)

The book tells you that you no longer need any emotional blocks and you feel them just melt away. The book shows you how to determine when you are full of the right foods for you and at that time you will want a glass of water. You will have no desire to eat extra food you will just drink the water. No desire to overeat. That desire just goes away as you sip your water. In fact any time you feel emotional stress you will drink water and that stress will melt away leaving you with no desire to overeat.

You feel very positive and relaxed as you turn to the next page of this magic book. The book now tells you how to speed up your metabolism to digest your food faster. It tells you the exact way that is right for you and your body. It also tells you how to eliminate your food faster. It tells you that in 15 minutes after you get up in the morning you will have a complete evacuation of food and waste from your body.

(Close your eyes for a moment and feel this information being absorbed.)

You are happy knowing that your emotional ties to eating have just disappeared. You are in control and controlling your emotions and your weight. Now close the book and smile and place it back in the book shelf. Look at the other end of the room. There is a table with a light directly over it. Lie down on the table and look up at the light. Watch as the light turns into electric blue light. This light is warm and peaceful and you feel peaceful when you look at the light. Feel this warm electric blue light come into your body and into your head.

Feel and Know that this beautiful blue light is healing any emotional issues that you attach to overeating. Making you positive and happy. Dispelling any negativity. Just making it go away. Feel this light inside your head changing all your negative patterns into positive ones. Lifting away all the negativity leaving only joyful, positive, happy thoughts. Feel the healing taking place right now, in this time, in this place.

As the electric blue light, this peaceful light enters your body and your mind. Feel how the blue light makes you think thin. Picture yourself in this blue light how you are meant to be at your ideal weight. See how you nicely your clothes fit, how happy your face is, how good your body looks. Feel your self-confidence. See how self-assured and in control of all your eating habits. Feel how happy you are. Know and trust that you will keep this image with you in your mind and that this image is becoming a reality right now.

(Close your eyes for a moment and feel this blue light.)

Now feel and watch as the electric blue light comes out of your mind and your body the same way it went in. Know that it takes with it all the negative behavior patterns, all the negative thoughts. Moving them out of your body and your mind. Leaving you peaceful, thinking thin and positive. Leaving the imprint in your mind of your ideal image filled with confidence and looking so well at your ideal weight.

Let's get up off the table feeling happy and walk out of the room and back to the stairs. Let's walk up the stairs.

Step 1 – Feeling good and full of energy.

Step 2 – Feeling positive.

Step 3 – So very Relaxed.

Step 4 – Happy.

Step 5 – Drinking water when you want to overeat.

Step 6 – No desire to Overeat.

Step 7 – Very Confident and very relaxed.

Step 8 – Picturing your ideal image in your mind.

Step 9 – In control of all your eating habits.

Step 10 – Feeling centered and whole in body, mind and spirit.

Now let's turn and walk back to the fireplace and sit back in the chair. See the fire in the fireplace. Feel the warmth of the fire. Smile knowing you are losing weight and in control of your goal. You are happy, filled with positive thoughts and peaceful. So very, very peaceful.

(Close your eyes for a moment and feel this feeling knowing that this feeling will stay with you.)

When you're ready, go to the next chapter.

CHAPTER SIX

BODY TRANSFORMATION

- ∞ Learn to Eat Slowly
- ∞ Stop Cravings and Hunger
- ∞ Control Overeating Effortlessly
- ∞ Naturally Select the Right Foods for You

We are what we eat. Many times our bodies crave certain foods, even though they are not good for us. This is because we are missing the correct vitamins, foods and nutrients that our body needs. We can stop cravings and hunger by taking the right vitamins and supplements. We also need to change how we eat and how much we eat. Choosing what we eat is important to get the body you want and maintain it for peak performance. Using the visualization in this Chapter, you will learn to select the right foods for you; control the amount you eat and eliminate cravings and hunger. But most important this visualization will help you transform your eating habits so that you can lose the weight.

So sit back and relax and get ready to lose weight!

CHANGING EATING HABITS VISUALIZATION

Intention: To Change Eating Habits

Find a comfortable place where you won't be disturbed and sit in a comfortable chair. Now sit back and relax with both feet on the floor and place your hands on the arm rests of the chair or in your lap—whichever is comfortable for you.

Concentrate as you breathe deeply letting the air come into your nose and out your mouth. Concentrate and breathe IN with the nose an OUT with the mouth. IN with the nose and OUT with the mouth. and IN with the nose and OUT with the mouth. Now let's concentrate on breathing OUT with the mouth and IN with the nose. And OUT with the mouth and IN with the nose. And OUT with the mouth and IN with the nose........

Imagine yourself sitting very relaxed by the ocean. It is night time and the stars are shining overhead. The temperature is exactly right for you. You are alone and you are peaceful. Hear the sounds of the waves coming to shore. Rhythmically, Softly. Feeling very relaxed in this peaceful place. Look up at the sky. You see one star that is brighter than the rest. Shining, twinkling so brightly. Watch as this star seems to come closer and closer to you. Feel the star's light. As the star gets closer to you it seems to send a pleasant sensation of warmth. Warm and relaxing.

(Close your eyes for a moment and feel the warmth as it gently relaxes you.)

Now watch as the star slowly recedes back to it's position in the sky and then back towards you again. It seems to be following a pattern. Very rhythmically. Coming closer, closer to you and then receding back to it's place in the sky. Feeling the star's warmth. Just watching the star move back and forth. Watching the star. As you continue to watch this moving star you seem to be getting more and more relaxed.

So very, very relaxed and peaceful and calm. Now watch as the star sends a gentle ray of light that surrounds your body. Softly, gently outlining your body.

The star's light is such a warm, pleasant sensation. You feel more and more relaxed. So safe. So peaceful. Now feel this warm sensation of star light enter into your forehead and as this warm, pleasant sensation enters your forehead all the lines in your forehead, all the tension seems to disappear. As this

warm sensation of starlight seems to take away all the tension. Now feel this warmth go into your eyes making them very, very heavy making you so relaxed. Feel how heavy your eyelids are as you're relaxing by the ocean, hearing the sounds of the sea and listening to the waves while you are getting deeper and deeper and even deeper relaxed. Feel and watch now as the warm, pleasant sensation of starlight goes into your throat and down into your chest, absorbing and taking away—all the tension, all the stress that is in your throat and chest area. Feel this warm sensation of starlight enter your abdominal area; your pelvic area and down your legs and into your feet. Taking away all the tension.

All the stress. Feeling deeper and deeper and even deeper relaxed as you listen to the waves of the sea. So relaxed as the tension and stress leave these areas of your body. The starlight, this warm sensation now goes to each and every toe and up the back of your leg and into your lower back. Absorbing all the tension and all the stress in the lower back area. Making you deeper, deeper and even deeper relaxed. This warm starlight sensation moves up your back and into all your internal organs of your body. Relaxing the stress, the tension in every fiber, every tissue, every organ of your body. Feel the soothing warm sensation go into your neck and shoulders. So much stress seems to go to this area but now you feel all this tension, all this stress just melts away as you get deeper and even deeper relaxed. As the tension in the neck, in the shoulders just releases and disappears.

Sitting on the shore, listening to the waves. How peaceful it is here. Feel the warm light go to the back of the head and inside the head making you feel deeper and deeper and even deeper relaxed.

As all the tension just melts away and you are feeling even deeper relaxed. More relaxed than you have ever known yourself to be.

(Close your eyes for a moment and feel how totally relaxed you are.)

Now stand up, taking this relaxing feeling with you and turn around. You see a beautiful house. This is your dream house. Walk up to the house and enter. The furniture in the house is so beautiful and to one side there is a spiral staircase. It goes up to a second level of the house. Let's go up the stairs feeling so very relaxed, very safe, very peaceful. As we go up the stairs, look at the pictures on the wall. How lovely they are. The carpet on the stairs is your favorite color. As you get to the top of the stair you see a room at the end of the hall. Walk up to the room and open the door. Inside the room is a very old antique mirror and as you walk up to it you know that this is a magic mirror.

Look into the mirror and see the image of who you are meant to be. You are the right weight, you have on the right clothes that fit so well, you have the right attitude. Look at the image in the mirror as it smiles back at you. Happy. Self-Confident. Joyful. The image is physically fit and healthy. You know you are this image in the mirror. Feeling very positive, turn around and look in back of you. There are two tables. On one table there is all the foods that are right for your body. There are fruits, vegetables, whole grains, lean meat and all the foods that are exactly right for your body.

(Close your eyes for a moment and see this good table of food.)

On the other table there are foods that are bad for your body; that harm your body; that stop you from being who you want to be. There may be breads, pastries, candy, soda and all the other foods that keep the weight on your body; all the foods that stop your body from working efficiently. Look down at your body. Look at the table with the bad foods. Knowing these foods make the body you are in.

(Close your eyes for a moment and imagine this bad table of food.)

Continue to look down at your body and then back at the table of bad foods. As you continue to do this you feel your desire for these foods just disappear. You no longer crave this food. You no longer want this food. This food that is wrong for you. That is keeping the weight on. That is stopping you from reaching your ideal weight. There is no desire for this food.

Look back at your image in the mirror. See and feel how happy you are at your ideal weight. Feel how nice your clothes fit, how happy you are at your ideal weight. Now look at the table of good foods. These are the foods that are right for you. The foods that will help you reach your ideal weight. They look so good. So filling. You desire these foods. You want these foods. Look back at the mirror and feel the joy at looking at the image of who you are. Look back at the table of good foods. These are the foods you need and want. Look over at the table of bad foods.

You don't want these foods. They won't even taste good to you anymore. You only want and need the good foods; the foods that are right for you. The good foods that give you energy, that taste so good. You desire these foods.

Look back at the image in the mirror and smile, knowing you only want the good foods for your body. Watch as the image smiles back. This image of who you are becoming, Right Now, In This Time, In this Place. You trust yourself and know that you only want and desire the good foods that make your body healthy. The good foods that make your body feel good and look good. The healthy foods that give your body the right nourishment it needs.

Go over to the good food table. There is a chair, sit down in this chair. It is so comfortable. There is a meal in front of you with all the right foods that you desire. The foods that you want and need. Watch as you pick up the utensils and start to eat. The food enters your mouth and tastes so good. You want to chew very, very slowly to get all the flavor of the food.

Each bite of the good food is chewed very, very slowly. Savoring the taste. It feels good to chew this food and not rush. You know that from now on you will chew your food very slowly. You have no more need to rush when you are eating.

(Close your eyes for a moment and see yourself chewing the food slowly.)

You will notice that when your body has had enough food to perform it's functions properly that you lose all the desire; all the need to eat any additional food. Eating smaller portions satisfies you. You want to eat smaller meals. It feels good to your body.

It feels good to eat less and enjoy every morsel of food chewing it so slowly. Watch as you drink some water. It tastes so good. So refreshing. This wonderful water. It taste so much better than any other drink. You like the taste of water better than any other drink. You want and desire water. If you have a choice of drinks, you will always select water.

You want to drink the amount of water that is good for your body. Feel how your body is reacting so positively to the right foods and the right amount of foods. Feel it burning up the fat. Making you lean. Giving you energy. Feel your digestion speeding up and absorbing all the nutrients. Balancing all the systems in your body. Normalizing the thyroid and hormonal systems. Every system in the body working efficiently in the exact right way for you to reach and maintain your goal. Helping you to lose the weight right now. No more cravings for food. No more hunger. Eating right. Eating just enough for your body to work at peak performance.

(Close your eyes for a moment. Feel and See your body working at peak performance.)

Feeling good and knowing that you will always continue to do what's right for your body, get up from the table. Turnaround now and look in the mirror. See yourself at your ideal weight and smile. You are this image in the mirror. You feel it. You know it. You trust it. You are happy and feel full of energy.

Keep this image in your mind as you walk out of the room. Remember this image as you walk down the stairs and out of the door. Now walk back to your place by the ocean and sit down. You feel so happy, so peaceful knowing you are losing weight. That you are becoming the person you are meant to be. The image in the mirror. The image in your mind. The image of you! Trusting that your body is doing what it needs to do. Feeling so relaxed and peaceful listening to the waves as they gently come into shore.

(Close your eyes for a moment and feel this feeling knowing that this feeling will stay with you.)

When you're ready, go to the next chapter.

CHAPTER SEVEN

EXERCISE MOTIVATION

- ∞ Learn the Joy of Exercise
- ∞ Find the Right Exercise for You
- ∞ Get the Desire to Exercise Regularly
- ∞ Make Your Body Feel as Good as it Looks

If you exercise a least thirty minutes a day, three times a week you will lose weight. Exercise is not only important for weight loss. It helps to keep our bodies healthy and balanced. Disease control and prevention, like osteoporosis and heart disease, can be aided by exercising. In fact, exercise can even help prevent premature death. Keeping all of our body's internal and external systems in good working order can be accomplished through exercise.

There are emotional benefit of exercise—it lifts the spirit. When you exercise it produces chemicals called endorphins. These endorphins calm and relax the body which helps fight stress, depression, anger and other emotional problems. It is said by many psychologists that if you take a long walk when you are depressed, the feeling of depression will lift. So you see exercise is an important factor to help you balance your body, mind and spirit.

The importance of exercise is well documented. However knowing what exercise is right for you and getting motivated to exercise regularly is another issue. The visualization in this chapter will help you discover what type of exercise is right for you. If you are extremely overweight you might want to check with your traditional or alternative doctor to find out what and how much exercise you should start out with. If the doctor suggests something different than the visualization, remember this is just the starting point and that you will be getting closer to your goal. Remember your mind and spirit are very powerful and by using visualization any goal can be actualized. Trust that your body will catch up and it will. Eventually you will be able to do any exercise that you want to.

In our busy lives we sometimes feel there isn't enough time to exercise. We need take responsibility and find the time because exercise fights stress. Remember stress is the primary cause of weight gain. To get motivated to exercise start with a positive attitude and think about how your mind, body and spirit will look and feel by exercising regularly. Then take action and set aside time and just do it.

Positive attitude and emotions help to empower you and keep up your motivation. Joy is one of the most powerful gifts that is provided to us to use as a tool for positive reinforcement. If you do something you like, you get a feeling of joy. Therefore, if you get joy every time you exercise you will stay motivated and exercise. The following visualization helps you find the right exercise, get joy when you exercise and gives you the desire to exercise to make your body feel as good as it looks. So sit back, relax and get ready to lose weight!

EXERCISE VISUALIZATION

Intention: To Get Motivated and Enjoy Exercise.

Find a comfortable place where you won't be disturbed and sit in a comfortable chair. Now sit back and relax with both feet on the floor and place your hands on the arm rests of the chair or in your lap—whichever is comfortable for you.

Concentrate as you breathe deeply letting the air come into your nose and out your mouth. Concentrate and breathe IN with the nose an OUT with the mouth. IN with the nose and OUT with the mouth. And IN with the nose and OUT with the mouth. Now let's concentrate on breathing OUT with the mouth and IN with the nose. And OUT with the mouth and IN with the nose. And OUT with the mouth and IN with the nose……..

Imagine you are walking down a city street. There is so much going on. See the people walking back and forth. Here the sounds of the cars and buses in the street. See how the sunlight reflects it's light off the tall buildings. You see a beautiful building before you. Walk into the Lobby. Look at the beautiful floors. The architecture. It is peaceful here. All the noise from the street has quieted down.

Look at the back of the lobby. You see a door there. Walk to the door. As you come closer to the door you see that your name is on it. Open the door and walk in. You see a soft comfortable bed. Go to the bed and lie down on it closing your eyes. It is so soft it feels like you are floating on a cloud.

In fact the bed becomes a cloud and starts to lift in the air. You are safe and peaceful and you like this weightless feeling. You feel so comfortable, so relaxed. It is so quiet here. Your mind slows down and your eyes become very, very heavy as you start to become more and more relaxed, just floating gently on this cloud. So peaceful. So relaxed.

It is so quiet here and you feel your mind relax more and more and more as you gently float.

(Close your eyes for a moment and see yourself floating on cloud.)

You feel your neck, your shoulders and your back just relax as you gently float on this soft, soft cloud. Your arms and hands just relax as you float on this cloud without a care or worry in the world. Feeling so safe, so relaxed. Just floating softly, gently.

Your legs and feet feel so relaxed now. In fact your whole body has never been more relaxed and as you float you feel this relaxation get deeper and deeper and even deeper. Just floating. Every part of your body and your mind becomes deeper and deeper relaxed as you float. Feeling so very, very relaxed. Now feel the cloud drifting back down towards the room and as you count backwards from 5 to 1 the cloud will get closer and closer to the room. You will feel more and more relaxed as you get deeper relaxed with every number.

5 – Deeper, Deeper.

4 – Even Deeper

3 – So relaxed

2 – Deeper, deeper and even deeper.

So relaxed and at the next number you will be more relaxed than you have ever known yourself to be.

Deep, deep relaxation – 1.

Sit up on the bed. Look to the left side of the room. There is a movie screen with a comfortable chair in front of it. Get up and sit in the chair. The room is quiet. Look at the movie screen. See the lights flicker on the screen. Focus on the screen. You see a flock of flying geese in a V formation. They are flying to their destination and as you watch these geese flying, you know that you are moving towards your destination of wanting and getting regular exercise. Just focus on the geese. There are no distractions. You feel your mind shifting towards wanting to exercise. Needing exercise. Desiring exercise. Enjoying exercise.

(Close your eyes for a moment and feel this feeling.)

Now watch as the geese fly off the screen and the screen becomes the most beautiful color you have ever seen. As you look into this color you see an image coming towards you. As the image gets closer you recognize that the image is You, physically fit, as you are meant to be. The image of you is exercising. It may be running, walking or playing a sport like basketball, tennis. Anything that feels right to you. You see yourself clearly. It could be at the gym—lifting weights, doing yoga, aerobics or working with machines. Whatever the exercise is -it becomes clear to you. It could even be a combination of different kinds of sports or exercise. Whatever it is, it is exactly right for you. The exercise that is right for your body to be healthy and physically fit.

(Close your eyes for a moment and see yourself doing the exercise that is right for you.)

Concentrate on the image of you doing this exercise. Feel the muscles working. Feel the strength. Feel the elation of your emotions as you continue to exercise. Without struggle. Just enjoying the exercise. Look at your face. You are smiling. You are happy. So joyful. Every time you exercise you will feel this joy. It fills you. Motivates you. You want to exercise to feel this joy. Look and see how you are accomplishing your perfect body. Your body in such good shape. Feeling good. Looking good. You like exercise. You need exercise. You want exercise. Feel the fat in your body just disappear as it is replaced with good, lean muscle tissue. You are winning! Feel the alertness of your mind. Your mental concentration is focused on exercise. Feel your inner power building and You Know you can accomplish anything you want. This power brings joy and motivation. You want this feeling. You want your body to look and feel good and you know that you are accomplishing this In This Time, In This Place, Right Now.

(Close your eyes for a moment and feel the joy and the power exercise brings you.)

Watch your image. Anytime you feel stress you will want to exercise. In fact you want to exercise at least thirty minutes a day, three times a week. You feel the energy and joy in your body when you exercise. You always find the time to exercise. There is always enough time for you to exercise. Your body feels so good. Your mind is alert. What a wonderful feeling! It feels so good to exercise. To be good at exercise. Without distractions. Exercise time for you is a special time. A time to bring your body-mind and spirit in balance.

A time to focus and center on yourself. To be One with yourself. Feeling positive and joyful in exercising. Feeling whole in body, mind and spirit.

Now watch as your image on the screen stops and looks at you. Look back at that image. Feel that image. This is You! Smile at your image and watch as it smiles back. Feel, Know and Trust that you will exercise regularly, that you feel joy at exercising, that you are good at exercise.

That you want to exercise and that this feeling will stay with you! The more you exercise, the better you will get at it. The more you will desire it.

Feel this. Know this. Trust this.

(Close your eyes for a moment and feel this feeling.)

Now watch as your image fades back into the screen. Get up from the chair and walk slowly to the door. With each step you take towards the door you have the desire to exercise. You feel the joy of exercise. You find time to exercise. You want to exercise. Walk through the door and into the lobby. You feel full of energy, so focused, so motivated and you are happy to know this feeling will stay with you.

And when you're ready, go to the next chapter.

CHAPTER EIGHT

STRESS RELIEVING MEDITATIONS

- ∞ Eliminate Stress on All Levels
- ∞ Eliminate Emotional and Nutritional Stress
- ∞ Eliminate Physical and Environmental Stress

Stress affects how we look, think and feel. It is the major culprit to weight gain. In fact, stress is produced by every reaction we have or every action that we perform. Stress may play a part in every illness or disease, as well as, affecting the balance of body chemistry.

Originally the body's method of handling excessive stress was the "fight or flight" response. When this response is triggered, adrenaline is pumped into the bloodstream and the sympathetic nervous system also releases a similar hormone into the body. More oxygen and sugar is then pumped into the blood. As this occurs breathing increases, senses sharpen, digestion stops and the muscles become tense. This usually happens for a short period of time. The stress in our lives has increased tremendously, even for our children, and I believe that we are in this "flight or fight" mode more often than we should be.

The down side to continually being in this "fight or flight" mode is that imbalances result in the body that paves the way for potential physical and emotional problems by eroding our immune system.

Let's take a look at what prolonged stress does. After our reaction to stress our body's go through a period of resistance before it gets exhausted. The weakest part of the body breaks down and causes imbalances in the body's system that cause weight gain, illness or emotional disturbances.

There are many books and methods to relieve stress. Relaxation is a proven method to reduce stress. Visualization is a form of relaxation. Combine this with the breathing method found in the visualization preparation, which activates the major quieting nerve of the body (The Vagus Nerve), and the Power of Intention and stress can be minimized or eliminated very effectively.

We already discussed that the four types of stress—Emotional, Nutritional, Physical and Environmental. Daily stress is as individualized as each person.

By using visualization as a tool, we can actually cope with and relieve stress on all four levels. The visualizations in this Chapter are short and effective. Each visualization releases stress on all levels or a particular type of stress. By selecting and using the correct visualization(s) daily or whenever you need them provides you two things: 1) you acknowledge the stress and 2) you can release it faster. The extra benefit is that by keeping a record of which stress(es) repeatedly are prevalent in your life you can take steps to minimize and/or eliminate them on other levels to gain a happier life.

STRESS VISUALIZATIONS "THE WATERFALL"

Intention: To Eliminate Stress on ALL Levels

Find a comfortable place where you won't be disturbed and sit in a comfortable chair. Now sit back and relax with both feet on the floor and place your hands on the arm rests of the chair or in your lap—whichever is comfortable for you.

Concentrate as you breathe deeply letting the air come into your nose and out your mouth. Concentrate and breathe IN with the nose an OUT with the mouth. IN with the nose and OUT with the mouth. And IN with the nose and OUT with the mouth. Now let's concentrate on breathing OUT with the mouth and IN with the nose. And OUT with the mouth and IN with the nose. And OUT with the mouth and IN with the

Imagine you are in a peaceful wooded spot. The sky is blue, the sun is shining. The smell of the flowers is so wonderful. Look to your right. You see a pool of water with a beautiful waterfall. This is your private place. No one can enter here. Take off your clothes and lay them on the soft green grass besides the pool. Walk into the water. The temperature is just right for you. Walk under the waterfall. Feel the water flowing gently over your body. So clean. So Fresh. Now watch as the water turns into multi-colored lights. The lights are so beautiful. Watch as the multi-colored lights turn into emerald green light.

Gently cascading around your body. This beautiful green light. Feel the light surround your body and enter into your body. This beautiful green healing light. Feel the green light go to every physical stress point in your body. Absorbing any physical stress, any pain, any tension. Absorbing it all away. Healing you. Healing your body. Relieving all the stress, the tension, the pain. Healing you right now, in this time, in this place. Making your body whole and healthy.

(Close your eyes for a moment and feel this emerald green light.)

Now watch as the emerald green light turns to electric blue light. Peaceful light. Feel this blue light enter into your body and your mind. Releasing negativity, Absorbing all the emotional stress, Healing your mind. This peaceful electric blue light shifting your mind, removing negative patterns. Making you whole and healthy in mind. Feeling so positive, so peaceful, so happy as this electric blue light heals your mind In This Time, In This Place, Right now.

(Close your eyes for a moment and feel this electric blue light.)

Now watch as this electric blue light turns to brilliant purple light. Spiritual light. Surrounding your body, entering into your body finding all the doubts, all the stress that stops you from reaching your goal. Feel it melt them away, this wonderful purple light. You are focused. You are centered. You feel loved and cherished in this wonderful, brilliant purple light.

You feel whole in spirit and your life has purpose and meaning.

(Close your eyes for a moment and feel this purple light.)

Now watch as this purple light turns to white light. Surrounding your body. Protecting you from negativity. Keeping all negative feelings away from you. This white light will stay with you. Protecting you. Keeping you stress free on all levels. Feel the happiness. Feel the joy. Feel the Peace. You are stress free in body, mind and spirit.

Feel it. Know It. Trust It.

(Close your eyes for a moment and feel this beautiful white light.)

Walk out of the pool and put on your clothes. Look over to the waterfall and know you are happy and positive and stress free in body, mind and spirit. This feeling will stay with you.

"THE OCEAN"

Intention: To Eliminate Emotional and Nutritional Stress

Find a comfortable place where you won't be disturbed and sit in a comfortable chair. Now sit back and relax with both feet on the floor and place your hands on the arm rests of the chair or in your lap—whichever is comfortable for you.

Concentrate as you breathe deeply letting the air come into your nose and out your mouth. Concentrate and breathe IN with the nose an OUT with the mouth. IN with the nose and OUT with the mouth. And IN with the nose and OUT with the mouth. Now let's concentrate on breathing OUT with the mouth and IN with the nose. And OUT with the mouth and IN with the nose. And OUT with the mouth and IN with the nose........

Imagine it is near dawn in the morning. You are at a secluded beach. Look at the sky, it is still dark and cloudless. Look at the stars shining and twinkling in the sky. Look out at the ocean. See the moon shining it's rays on the water. Watch as the waves come crashing in to shore. One after the other. Feel the power of the waves. See the foam. Feel the spray of the waves. You are an expert swimmer. Walk into the water facing the waves. Feel the undertow of the waves making it difficult for you to stand on your feet. You sway as the waves crash into you but you do not fall down. Keep walking into the waves. Deeper and deeper into the waves. Feel the waves as they hit you.

Turn and face sideways to your left, making it easier to cut through the waves as they crash into you. Feel the power of the waves.

Turn to your right side and continue to cut deeper into the waves as they continue to crash with full force into you, one after another, after another. You are getting further and further out. Turn and dive into the next wave. Feel the power around you as you dive through the wave coming out on the other side.

Swim into the waves until you get to the place where the waves start. The place where the gentle swells that are not yet waves roll and rock you gently. Rest and float on your back. Feel the peace and serenity as you float on your back looking up at the sky.

(Close your eyes for a moment and feel this peace and serenity.)

Watch as the sky changes colors. See dawn breaking in the sky as the colors splash across it. Be still and serene as you watch the sun come up and feel the rays of the sun shining down on you making you strong. Taking away all the emotional stress, all the negativity that is stopping you from reaching your goal. Taking away all the nutritional stress in your body. These wonderful warm rays of sunlight as you float gently rocking back and forth. Healing you. Soothing you. Feeling so happy and full of energy. When you are ready swim out of the ocean and stand on the shore. Look out over the ocean. You are dried and warmed by the sun. You are strong and at peace.

This feeling will stay with you.

"THE HEALING POOL"

Intention: To Eliminate Physical and Environmental Stress

Find a comfortable place where you won't be disturbed and sit in a comfortable chair. Now sit back and relax with both feet on the floor and place your hands on the arm rests of the chair or in your lap—whichever is comfortable for you.

Concentrate as you breathe deeply letting the air come into your nose and out your mouth. Concentrate and breathe IN with the nose an OUT with the mouth. IN with the nose and OUT with the mouth. And IN with the nose and OUT with the mouth. Now let's concentrate on breathing OUT with the mouth and IN with the nose. And OUT with the mouth and IN with the nose. And OUT with the mouth and IN with the nose........

Imagine you are in a meadow. The sun is shining and it is peaceful. Look at the green grass, the flowers, the trees, the clear blue sky.

To your right you see a pool of water. It is tranquil and serene. See the clean, clear water sparkling in the sun. You are alone and this is your special place. No one can enter. Take off your clothes and step into the water. Feel the water warm on your feet and ankles as you wade in. Sit down in the water, it is not deep. Feel the water embrace your thighs, stomach, shoulders, neck. You are immersed in the water. Look down and see the soft white mud.

Touch the mud and feel how warm and soothing it is. Feel the tension float away as you relax in the water. You are comfortable. Feel the mud surround each joint, each muscle in the body. Feel the white mud going into your body. Imagine that the mud is drawing all the toxins, all the pain away from every fiber, every muscle, every bone and every tissue in your body.

(Close your eyes for a moment and imagine this wonderful, warm white mud.)

The white mud just absorbing it away. All the physical stress in your body just disappears making your body stress free. Feel all the stress just rain away into the mud as you relax and know you are healing. Now watch as the mud comes out of the body the same way it went in.

(Close your eyes for a moment and imagine the white mud.)

When you are done wash the remaining mud off of your body. Stand up and step out of the pool. Lay down on the soft green grass and look up at the sky. The sun is warm and shining as it dries you off. Feel the warm tones of blue and green light emit from the sun and surround your body, healing it now. Your body is free of pain, free of stress.

(Close your eyes for a moment and feel your body free of pain and stress.)

Sit up and stretch your body and feel how good it feels. Stand up and put on your clothes. You are comfortable. You are at peace. This feeling will stay with you.

CHAPTER NINE

THIN MEDITATIONS

- ∞ Learn to Think Thin
- ∞ Lose Weight Naturally
- ∞ Maintain Weight Loss

Learning to think thin is an important part of weight loss. The term "You are What You Eat" applies to the body just as "You Are What You Think" applies to the mind. By reinforcing the thought of Being Thin we boost our minds to effect weight loss on a physical level. This helps to change negative thought patterns and negative programming into positive ones. The Thought is very powerful. Everything is comprised of energy. Energy has power. Thought is an energy form and therefore it has power.

By thinking thin you are harnessing this thought form energy to self-empower yourself to help you reach your goal. Circumstances can not keep you from attaining your goals but negative thought can. It sets up a resistance in your mind-body-spirit connection that holds you back. By constantly using positive thought to think thin you slowly change your belief system and it becomes imprinted in your mind that indeed you are thin. Once this imprint is in your mind, your body responds by losing weight. Our minds are so powerful and visualization is a tool to harness the power of the mind. The visualizations in this chapter are short and very powerful. They will keep you thinking thin and help you become thin.

So sit back, relax and get ready to lose weight!

THIN VISUALIZATIONS
"THE DOWNWARD STAIRCASE"

Intention: To Lose Weight!

Find a comfortable place where you won't be disturbed and sit in a comfortable chair. Now sit back and relax with both feet on the floor and place your hands on the arm rests of the chair or in your lap—whichever is comfortable for you.

Concentrate as you breathe deeply letting the air come into your nose and out your mouth. Concentrate and breathe IN with the nose an OUT with the mouth. IN with the nose and OUT with the mouth. And IN with the nose and OUT with the mouth. Now let's concentrate on breathing OUT with the mouth and IN with the nose. And OUT with the mouth and IN with the nose. And OUT with the mouth and IN with the nose........

Imagine you are on a winding path in the woods. You are walking down this path. See the soft dirt beneath your feet. The green grass and trees along side the path. As you turn around the corner of the path you see a house. It is most beautiful house you have ever seen. The doors. The windows. Walk up to the door and walk in. There is a staircase to your right. The staircase is different. It is a magic staircase. You know that as you walk down these steps you will be losing weight. At each and every step that you go down you will be losing weight. You will feel the weight coming off your body. What a wonderful place! Walk over to the staircase and look down. There are 10 steps and they are covered in your favorite carpet. At the bottom of the stairs you see a floor to ceiling mirror. You can watch yourself in the mirror as you are walking down the steps.

(Close your eyes for a moment and see yourself in the mirror.)

Let's walk down the steps. As I count down from 10 to 1 you will feel more and more relaxed. You will be watching yourself in the mirror losing weight as you go down each step.

At every step more weight will come off. Take a breath and let's begin.

(After each step close your eyes for a moment and notice the changes taking place in your body as the weight comes off.)

Step 10 – Look in the Mirror. See the weight start to come off your body. Feel the weight come off.

Step 9 – Feeling more relaxed watch as even more weight comes off your body. Watch as your clothes shrink to fit your body that losing weight right now.

Step 8 – Watch in the Mirror. Weight disappears. Feel your emotional stress, your physical stress leave your body. As you lose weight in this time.

Step 7 – Feel More weight come off your body as the desire for the wrong foods just goes away. As the desire to overeat just disappears as the weight disappears from your body.

Step 6 – Feeling so relaxed as more and more weight comes off. Look in the mirror. See how thin you are. Know how thin you are.

Step 5 – More and more and more weight comes off as you know you are releasing all emotional ties to eating. All the negative behavior patterns disappear as you watch yourself losing weight, stepping down the stairs, looking in the mirror.

Step 4 – Feel and watch as more weight comes off your body. Run your hands down your body and feel how slender you are. Look in the mirror and see how slender you are.

Step 3 – Concentrate and feel your body's metabolism burning away the fat. How all the systems in your body are working correctly and at peak performance. Digesting the food, balancing the hormonal levels, giving you energy, taking the weight off.

Step 2 – Feeling so happy at all the weight you are losing. Desiring only the right foods for you. Feeling peaceful as you see more weight come off your body. The pounds just melting away.

Step 1 – Watch as you reach your ideal weight. The weight you are meant to be. All the weight gone. Thinking thin. Being Thin. Feeling energy. Feeling Happy. Feeling centered.

> Walk over to the mirror. Smile at your image. This IS YOU! Look at the weight you have lost. Feeling good and knowing you have accomplished much this day—Smile and feel contentment. This feeling will stay with you.

"THE WEIGHT LOSS SAUNA"

Intention: To Lose Weight!

Find a comfortable place where you won't be disturbed and sit in a comfortable chair. Now sit back and relax with both feet on the floor and place your hands on the arm rests of the chair or in your lap—whichever is comfortable for you.

Concentrate as you breathe deeply letting the air come into your nose and out your mouth. Concentrate and breathe IN with the nose an OUT with the mouth. IN with the nose and OUT with the mouth. And IN with the nose and OUT with the mouth. Now let's concentrate on breathing OUT with the mouth and IN with the nose. And OUT with the mouth and IN with the nose. And OUT with the mouth and IN with the nose........

Imagine you are in your favorite room. You feel so relaxed. Your favorite things are all around you. In one corner of the room you see a door. As you walk up to the door you see it is a Sauna. This is your private place. You are alone and none will disturb you. Take off your clothes and walk into the sauna shutting the door. It smells of Eucalyptus and cedar and is so aromatic. The temperature is warm but right for you. Look to your left. There is a bench with big soft towels on it. Pick up a towel. On your right are three levels of long wooden seats. The seats are long enough to lie down on. Know that the first level will be hot, the second level even hotter and the third level that is closest to the ceiling will be the hottest.

Choose a level and place the towel down. Find the level that is right for you. Lie down and feel the heat permeate your body.

Feel the heat relieving all the stress, all the tension in every fiber, every bone and every muscle in your body.

(Close your eyes and feel the warm relaxing heat.)

Feeling so warm and so relaxed. Look to your right. In the corner is a white light. Feel this white light come into your body. It is a pleasant feeling. Feel the white light taking away all the negativity, all the emotional stress, releasing all your emotional ties to eating. Absorbing them away from your body and your mind. Making them just disappear.

(Close your eyes for a moment and imagine this white light.)

Now feel the heat of the Sauna as it is melting away the pounds. Just letting them melt away as the white light soothes you, relaxes you—taking away the desire to overeat. Making this desire just disappear leaving you wanting water whenever you desire to overeat. This desire for food will just go away as you sip your water. The water you want instead of the desire for food. And the heat of the sauna is just melting away the pounds, one by one. Making you lose the weight that is right for you for this day. Feel the weight coming off. Know that the weight is coming off. Trust that the weight is coming off.

(Close your eyes and feel the weight coming off your body.)

Feel the white light healing any part of your mind, your body, your spirit, that needs support and healing. Healing everything that is stopping you from being who you want to be. Feel the peace. Feel the happiness.

(Close your eyes for a moment and feel this happiness.)

Get up off the seat. Open the door and walk into the room. With each step you take towards the door, you know you are becoming thinner, more vibrant and full of energy. Smile because you know you are losing weight and open the door and step into the room. Remembering this wonderful feeling that will stay with you.

"THE PERFECT BODY"

Intention: To Lose Weight!

Find a comfortable place where you won't be disturbed and sit in a comfortable chair. Now sit back and relax with both feet on the floor and place your hands on the arm rests of the chair or in your lap—whichever is comfortable for you.

Concentrate as you breathe deeply letting the air come into your nose and out your mouth. Concentrate and breathe IN with the nose an OUT with the mouth. IN with the nose and OUT with the mouth. And IN with the nose and OUT with the mouth. Now let's concentrate on breathing OUT with the mouth and IN with the nose. And OUT with the mouth and IN with the nose. And OUT with the mouth and IN with the nose........

Imagine you are standing in front of a mountain. There is a cave in front of you. You feel safe and relaxed. Walk into the cave. At the back of the cave you see a wall of clear white crystal. Walk over to the white crystal wall. It is sparkling with light. Look up. You see a hole in the cave's ceiling where sunlight is coming through. It is lighting up the crystal wall. Look back at the crystal wall and as you do you see your image in the crystal. Watch as your image starts to change. As you watch you can feel the changes happening inside your body. You see your body shrinking to the weight you want to be. You feel the fat in your body turn to lean muscle tissue. You see and feel yourself shrinking down to your perfect weight, your ideal weight. Your clothes fit so well.

Your muscles are becoming defined. You feel strong. You feel healthy. Watch. Watch as your body becomes your perfect body. The body that is right for you. Feel it happening. See the changes taking place. Feel the changes taking place in your body.

(Close your eyes for a moment and feel this happening.)

Every muscle, every bone, every tissue, every fiber in your body shifting to perfection. To perfect working order. Your body perfect in every way. Feeling strong and physically fit. All the systems in your body working correctly and efficiently. Watch as the sunlight reflects off the crystal wall as the crystal light reflects into your body. Helping the changes to manifest right here, in this time, in this place. Making you whole in body, mind and spirit. Creating your perfect body. Now look at the crystal wall and see your perfect body. Look down at your body and see that your body is perfect in every way. Touch your body and feel the difference. See the difference. Know that the changes have happened. You feel centered, full of energy, powerful. Full of joy.

(Close your eyes for a moment and imagine touching your body and feeling the difference.)

Feel how it feels to be in your perfect body. Anytime there is stress you will see your perfect body. Anytime you need motivation you will feel this perfect body.

Anytime a negative situation appears you will see your perfect body and any negativity will just go away. You will remember this feeling of your perfect body. Keeping this feeling with you, turn and walk out of the cave.

You are happy and content in your perfect body. You are motivated and know that you are creating your perfect body right now. Smile and hold onto this feeling.

EPILOGUE

Visualization helps you to manifest your goals. It creates an awareness of yourself and allows you to admit *and* maintain your own personal power. Using positive thought through visualization can cause the expected changes designed by your "Intent" to occur.

Approach visualization with the certainty of what you want to accomplish and why you want to accomplish it and then let the visualization provide the means to that accomplishment. When doing a visualization make sure you are clear and focused on your Intent. Feel, Know and Trust that your physical body will respond and it will!

Remember visualization works through repetition so keep at it and you will manifest the body, mind and spirit that you are meant to be.

Good Luck and Much Success to you. I know you will lose weight!

—Linda Mackenzie

BONUS SECTION

'LindaMac' Diet

It was 1989 when it happened. I got the Epstein Barr Virus. This was at a time when the medical community doubted its very existence. There was no known treatment. As a sole-supported single Mom, with a daughter getting ready for college, I could not afford to be sick.

Thus it was the start of a three year journey into the study of alternative medicine. I used a combination of hypnotherapy, herbs, supplements, vitamins, lifestyle and the following 'LindaMac' diet. The diet specifically helps my body to maintain a high immune system. The result short term was that I lost weight, Then, over a period of time – I healed myself. I am still on this diet today.

Wanting to help people in the discovery of self-healing techniques I became a Clinical Hypnotherapist and President of a dietary vitamin and supplement manufacturing company. I then lectured at hospitals and conferences all over the United States for the next several years.

One of the most valuable things that I found in my healing experience was my change in diet. I had never realized before the Epstein Barr Virus episode that "you are what you eat" is just as important as "you are what you think." That food can help you heal. Diet is particularly important because the kinds of foods you eat can actually help boost your immune system. This can aid you to fight disease and minimize or eliminate its symptoms.

The diet I ultimately adopted—for life—makes me feel good, keeps my immune system high so that I rarely get sick and actually keeps me looking younger than I actually am.

I can remember being asked to a pre-screening by my good friend, and Golden Globe winner, actress Sally Kirkland. The screening was of a motion picture by the late John Daly, who was a delightful man. I remember coming out of the elevator and people were gravitating towards me. The audience, made up mostly of both young and old actors, actresses and students, were the beautiful people. Being average looking and not an actress I kept wondering why these people were giving me second looks. So I started looking back into them, not at them. Most looked stressed. They had an unhealthy patina to their skin. It was then I realized that what they were looking at, was not my face or body, it was my health. Being healthy does give out an aura that surrounds you and I was never more conscious of it than at that moment. I also realized that my diet was a key factor in creating that aura of health.

So with my healthy aura and youthful appearance created by my diet – I should be ecstatically happy right? Well, quite frankly I wasn't. There was a missing piece to the equation. I was on, what I called, the 'Linda-Mac' diet.

All my life I was an excellent cook. My grandfather was a top Italian chef in New York City's major hotels. My uncles were chefs and my father, well, he was a cook in the army. My mother could boil spaghetti, and with water still in the pot—burn it. So needless to say, by a very young age, I joined my father in preparing most of the meals for our family out of a need for taste and, sorry Mom, survival. Taste was a very important part of my life and a sense I rarely took for granted.

As I got older, my family and friends looked forward to eating whatever I concocted in my kitchen, then came the Epstein Barr Virus and the 'LindaMac' diet. I was so limited in the foods that I was eating, which lacked texture and taste, that it led me on a 20 year journey to find a way to improve the taste of the 'LindaMac' diet.

Finally, I am back! My family and friends once again look forward to dining in my home. Most times they don't realize that they are participating in my 'LindaMac' diet and getting healthy by default. In this bonus section I have also included SUBSTITUTION TABLES so you can convert almost any recipe into the 'LindaMac' diet.

Everybody's body is different and I believe that no one should give up the power or responsibility of their own health. Working as a partner with your medical professionals, whether traditional or alternative, is your optimum method to achieving and maintaining your health. Be aware of how your body is responding to your medical treatments and never be afraid to question, question, question! Remember the responsibility of your body is yours and yours alone.

My 'LindaMac' diet consists of foods that may help support the immune system and your weight loss goals, but because your body is unique—you and your body will have to decide what is right for you. Just remember, you have to really listen to your body. Your body will tell you whether or not they like the food you are eating, usually within twenty minutes after eating it. If your pulse is racing or you feel light headed or get a foggy feeling – maybe your food is the culprit. Test each food individually and see if you get the same reaction.

With my 'LindaMac' diet, which is similar to a Candida diet, you can try it for six weeks. Then try adding in different foods, one at a time, to see how your body reacts to them.

Can the 'LindaMac' diet work for both health and weight loss? I have been on this diet since 1992. At '70-something' I an on no medication, not even aspirin. Most people my age take 5-7 medications on average. The plus side of the 'LindaMac' diet is I am almost never sick, haven't had a major illness and I am, in perfect health in mind, body and spirit. Apart from the diet, I exercise with weights, aerobics and yoga, 1 hour a day, 5X a week. Since I am still a size 6, and look at least 15 years younger (without major plastic surgery) I know it's working for me. Here's hoping it works for you!

The 'LindaMac' Diet

Diet should be used for a minimum of 6 weeks. Then add foods back into the diet one by one and test your reaction to each one. I highly recommend sticking closely to the diet for the rest of your life.

NO LIST
Dairy (milk, yogurt, cheese, cream cheese),
Salt
Sugar
Wheat (whole wheat, white flour, kamut, amaranth, spelt)
Citrus Fruits, apples, pears, grapes
Prepared Foods with preservatives, food colorings, flavorings, dyes
Yeast
Caffeine (coffee, decaf coffee, tea or cola)
Alcohol
Carbonated Water, soda or drinks
Vinegar or Fermented foods
Leftovers (unless immediately frozen)
No raw vegetables or salads (except: 1 small salad 1X a week), potatoes, tomatoes, eggplant, mushrooms, iceberg lettuce
peanuts or pistachios
trout, orange roughy

YES LIST

Dairy: ONLY eggs, butter

Fruit: ONLY bananas, kiwi, pineapple, mango, guava, papaya, lemons, (after 6 weeks: blueberries, raspberries, blackberries)

Rice, Nuts and Grains: ONLY brown rice, quinoa and all nuts; except those on the No List

Pastas: ONLY Rice, Corn or Quinoa Pasta

Vegetables: All; 1 small raw salad a week, except those on the NO list

Meats and Poultry: ONLY beef, lamb, veal, venison, chicken, duck, pheasant and turkey

Fish: All; except those on the NO list

Sweeteners: ONLY Brown rice syrup (after 6 weeks: honey, molasses, maple syrup)

Beverages: ONLY Filtered Water, herbal teas

Breads: ONLY corn tortillas (after 6 weeks brown rice bread, 100% rye, no yeast or wheat)

Cooking Oils: ONLY olive oil or clarified butter

THE ABC'S OF SUBSTITUTION

The chart that follows is what I call The ABCs of Substitution. After over 25 years of experimenting, they seem to work virtually in every recipe that I can concoct or convert. In some cases I have given you several alternatives for the same item. Depending on your allergy sensitivities and your taste buds, it is totally up to you to select what substitution you may want to use.

Category	For Every:	Substitute	Uses and Amounts
Binders	1 cup of flour	Xantham Gum	Cakes: ½ Teaspoon Cookies: ¼ Teaspoon Muffins: ¾ Teaspoon
Xantham Gum in baked goods helps to bind and keep the ingredients together. It makes baked goods less crumbly and gives a better texture.			
Cooking Oil	1 Tablespoon Vegetable, Soy Bean or Canola Based Oil	Sunflower Oil	1 Tablespoon
	1 Tbs. Vegetable, Soy Bean or Canola Based Oil	Safflower Oil	1 Tablespoon
	1 Tbs. Vegetable, Soy Bean or Canola Based Oil	Olive Oil or Grapeseed Oil	1 Tablespoon
	1 Tbs. Vegetable, Soy Bean or Canola Oil	Melted Butter	1 Tablespoon
	1 Tbs. Vegetable Shortening	Organic Palm Oil Shortening	1 Tablespoon
Some people are allergic to soybean oil, canola oil (modified rapeseed plant) or conventional vegetable shortening (which is made with soybean oil) and they may be genetically modified. Canola oil may lose its healthy properties when heated and real butter may help the heart and have other benefits.			
Chocolate	1 sq. (1 oz.) chocolate	Carob Powder	3-4 Tablespoons
	1 cup Chocolate Chips	1 cup Carob Chips	1 Tablespoon
Eating 1.oz 75% dark chocolate a day may show benefits to heart health because of antioxidants called Flavanols—watch out for the fats and calories!			

Category	For Every:	Substitute	Uses and Amounts
Dairy	1 cup Cow's Milk	Rice Milk	1 cup less 2 Tablespoons
	1 cup Cow's Milk	Goats Milk	1 cup
	1 cup Buttermilk	Lemon Milk	Add 1 Tablespoon lemon juice to 1 cup minus 2 Tbs. rice milk
	1 cup Buttermilk	Apple Cider Milk	Add 1 Tablespoon apple cider vinegar to 1 cup minus 2 Tbs. rice milk
	1 whole Egg	Egg Yolk	2 Egg Yolks

Some say that if the whole egg is eaten, the albumen (white of the egg) counteracts the cholesterol in the egg yolk.

Pasta	Wheat	Quinoa Rice Corn Lentil Chickpea	Follow directions on package

My favorite is Quinoa pasta. It is more nutritious than whole milk and tastes the most like wheat pasta.

Salt	Iodized Salt	Sea Salt	

Sea salt tends to include naturally present trace minerals, such as iodine, magnesium, and potassium, which give sea salt a fresher, lighter flavor than standard table salt.

Flour	1 cup White	Home-made Wheat-Free Flour*	1 cup
	1 cup Whole Wheat		
	1 cup Kamut		
	1 cup Spelt		
	1 cup Amaranth		

Although they may process in the body differently Kamut, Amaranth and Spelt are still forms of wheat.

*Recipe for Home-made Wheat-Free Flour (Makes 4 ¾ cups)
    2 ½ cup Brown Rice Flour
    1 ¼ cup Cornstarch*
    ¾ cup Tapioca Flour
    ¼ cup White Rice Flour
Sift together ingredients. Store in airtight container in refrigerator.

*You can substitute Arrowroot Powder for Cornstarch

Sugar	1 cup White Sugar	Maple Syrup	¾ cup
	1 cup White Sugar	Honey	¾ cup
	1 cup Brown Sugar	Molasses	1 cup

Grade B Maple Syrup has more nutrients and Honey is the sweetest in recipes.

Other Books by Linda Mackenzie

Inner Insights - The Book of Charts
How to Self-Publish and Market Your Personal Growth Book
Help Yourself Heal with Self-Hypnosis
Symbols of You - A Self-Discovery Reference Guide

Audios by Linda Mackenzie

Total Mind-Body-Spirit Weight Loss Program
Help Yourself Heal - Menopause

Videos by Linda Mackenzie

Many Faces of Psychic Ability

Linda Mackenzie Websites

www.lindamackenzie.net
www.healthylife.net
www.HRNradio.com

www.ingramcontent.com/pod-product-compliance
Lightning Source LLC
LaVergne TN
LVHW010552070526
838199LV00063BA/4950